SARCOIDOSIS MANAGEMENT DIET COOKBOOK

Delicious Recipes For Optimal Health:

Boost Your Immunity With Balanced

Meals:

Enjoy Tasty Dishes For Better Well-

Being

DR. SHAYLA LEWIS

Table of Contents

DISCLAIMER

Write a brief complete Disclaimer for my diet cook book telling them that the author is not in any association with any company, business or individual and also this book is written by the authors knowledge and understanding

The information provided in this diet cookbook is based on the author's personal knowledge and understanding. The author is not affiliated with, endorsed by, or associated with any company, business, or individual. The recipes and dietary advice contained within this book are intended for informational purposes only. Readers should consult with a healthcare professional or a registered dietitian before making any significant changes to their diet or lifestyle. The author assumes no responsibility for any adverse effects that may result from the use or misuse of the information contained in this book.

CHAPTER ONE

Overview of Sarcoidosis and Its Effect on Health

Sarcoidosis is a multisystem inflammatory illness that can affect almost every organ in the body, however, it is most typically found in the lungs and lymph nodes.

The specific etiology of sarcoidosis is unknown, however, it is thought to be an aberrant immunological response to unknown environmental triggers in genetically predisposed individuals.

Sarcoidosis has a wide range of effects on health, from modest symptoms that resolve on their own to persistent and devastating problems. Sarcoidosis can sometimes cause irreparable organ damage, resulting in long-term issues such as lung fibrosis, eye difficulties, cardiac arrhythmias, and neurological impairment.

Sarcoidosis must be managed holistically, addressing both the underlying inflammation and the related symptoms. While corticosteroids and immunosuppressants are frequently prescribed to reduce inflammation and manage symptoms, lifestyle changes, including dietary interventions, are critical in optimizing health outcomes and improving the quality of life for people with sarcoidosis.

Diet is important in alleviating symptoms

Dietary interventions can have a major impact on the progression of sarcoidosis by reducing inflammation, boosting immunological function, and improving general health and well-being. While there is no "sarcoidosis diet," selecting smart dietary choices can help relieve symptoms, reduce inflammation, and promote the body's natural healing processes.

Certain foods and nutrients have been demonstrated to have anti-inflammatory characteristics, which may aid in reducing the inflammatory response associated with sarcoidosis. These include fruits, vegetables, whole grains, lean proteins, healthy fats, and diets high in antioxidants and phytonutrients. Processed foods, refined sugars, saturated fats, and high sodium intake, on the other hand, might aggravate inflammation and worsen symptoms.

Individuals with sarcoidosis can improve their overall health and quality of life by eating a balanced and nutritious diet rich in whole, unprocessed foods and limiting inflammatory triggers.

Components of a Sarcoidosis-Friendly Diet

A sarcoidosis-friendly diet should include nutrient-dense foods that boost immune function, reduce inflammation, and improve general health.

Fruits and vegetables are high in vitamins, minerals, antioxidants, and fiber, and should be the foundation of a sarcoidosis-friendly diet. Aim for a diversity of colors to ensure a wide range of nutrients.

Whole Grains: To maximize fiber and nutrient content, choose whole grains such as brown rice, quinoa, oats, and whole wheat bread instead of refined grains.

Lean Proteins: To support muscle health and repair, consume lean protein sources such as poultry, fish, beans, lentils, tofu, and tempeh.

Healthy Fats: Include sources of healthy fats like avocados, nuts, seeds, and olive oil, which are anti-inflammatory and promote cardiovascular health.

Antioxidant-Rich Foods: To battle oxidative stress and inflammation, eat foods strong in antioxidants including berries, leafy greens, nuts, seeds, and colorful fruits and vegetables.

Hydration: Drink enough water throughout the day to maintain good health and organ function.

Moderate salt and Sugar Consumption: Limit your intake of processed foods, which are generally heavy in salt and refined sugars, as excessive consumption can cause inflammation and increase the risk of chronic disease.

Individuals with sarcoidosis can better control their symptoms by prioritizing nutrient-rich diets and reducing inflammatory triggers.

Carbohydrates, antioxidants, and anti-inflammatory foods have important roles in managing sarcoidosis and promoting general health.

carbs: Choose complex carbs like whole grains, fruits, vegetables, and legumes, which provide long-term energy and fiber while reducing blood sugar spikes. Avoid processed carbohydrates and sugary snacks, which can cause inflammation and worsen symptoms.

Antioxidants are substances that help neutralize damaging free radicals in the body, thereby lowering oxidative stress and inflammation. Antioxidant-rich foods include berries, dark leafy greens, nuts, seeds, and colorful fruits and vegetables. Incorporating these foods into your diet can help protect against oxidative stress and improve immunological function.

Anti-Inflammatory Foods: Certain foods have been demonstrated to have anti-inflammatory characteristics, which can help regulate the inflammatory response associated with sarcoidosis. These include omega-3-rich seafood (such as salmon, mackerel, and sardines), turmeric, ginger, green tea, and foods high in monounsaturated fats, such as olive oil and avocado. Incorporating these anti-inflammatory foods into your diet will help reduce inflammation and alleviate sarcoidosis symptoms.

Grocery Shopping and Meal Planning Tips: Grocery shopping and meal planning are critical parts of managing sarcoidosis through nutrition. Here are some pointers to help you make smart food decisions and plan nutritious meals:

Create a Shopping List: Before going to the grocery store, develop a list of the goods you'll need depending on your meal plan and dietary preferences. This can help you stay focused and prevent making impulsive purchases of harmful meals.

Shop the Perimeter: Stick to the perimeter of the grocery store, where fresh produce, lean proteins, dairy, and whole grains are usually found. Limit your time spent in the aisles, where processed and packaged goods are typically exhibited.

Read product labels and ingredient lists to find hidden sources of extra sugars, bad fats, and artificial additives. Select items with few ingredients and avoid those with lengthy lists of chemicals and preservatives.

Bulk purchases of essential commodities such as grains, beans, nuts, and seeds can help you save money and reduce packaging waste. To preserve their freshness, store these goods in sealed containers.

Plan Balanced Meals: When preparing meals, aim for a mix of lean protein, whole grains, fruits and vegetables, and healthy fats. Experiment with new recipes and flavors to make meals more interesting and pleasurable.

Preparation Ahead: Use downtime to wash and cut veggies, marinate proteins, and cook grains and legumes. This will simplify meal preparation on hectic weekdays and make healthy eating more accessible.

Stay Flexible: Your meal plan should be adaptable to shifting schedules, cravings, and ingredient availability. Don't be hesitant to try new foods and dishes to keep your meals interesting and satisfying.

By following these grocery shopping and meal planning ideas, you may make the process of managing sarcoidosis through nutrition easier and more fun, while also improving your general health and well-being.

Essential Nutrients for Sarcoidosis Management: Sarcoidosis is a disorder in which granulomas grow in numerous organs, most notably the lungs and lymph nodes. Sarcoidosis management necessitates a holistic strategy, which includes nutritional considerations. Individuals with sarcoidosis benefit greatly from essential nutrients, which help to boost the immune system, reduce inflammation, and promote general health. These nutrients include vitamins, minerals, and antioxidants, as well as macronutrients like proteins, carbs, and fats.

Exploring Key Nutrients for Healing and Symptom Management: Specific nutrients have been discovered to have the ability to promote healing and reduce sarcoidosis symptoms. For example, antioxidants such as vitamin C, vitamin E, and beta-carotene can help lower oxidative stress and inflammation in the body.

Fish oil contains omega-3 fatty acids, which have anti-inflammatory effects and may benefit people with sarcoidosis, especially those who are experiencing lung inflammation. Furthermore, vitamin D is essential for immune function and bone health, and insufficiency is common in sarcoidosis patients, making supplementation or adequate sun exposure necessary.

CHAPTER TWO

A well-balanced diet high in vitamins, minerals, and micronutrients is critical for sarcoidosis treatment. Incorporating a mix of fruits, vegetables, whole grains, lean meats, and healthy fats into your meals ensures that you obtain a full range of nutrients. For example, colorful fruits and vegetables are high in vitamins A, C, and E, as well as antioxidants such as lycopene and beta-carotene. Fish, poultry, tofu, and beans are high in lean proteins, which are needed for tissue repair and immunological function. Whole grains such as quinoa, brown rice, and oats include complex carbs, fiber, and a variety of vitamins and minerals.

Sarcoidosis patients should prioritize nutrient-dense foods in their diets to meet their nutritional requirements. Some excellent sources of important nutrients are:

Lean proteins include fish, poultry, tofu, lentils, nuts, and seeds.

Fruits and vegetables include berries, citrus, leafy greens, tomatoes, sweet potatoes, and broccoli.

Whole grains include quinoa, brown rice, oats, barley, and whole wheat.

Healthy fats include avocados, olive oil, nuts, seeds, and fatty seafood such as salmon and mackerel.

Low-fat milk, yogurt, cheese, or fortified plant-based alternatives can provide calcium and vitamin D.

While there are basic criteria for recommended daily allowances (RDAs) of nutrients, individual requirements may differ depending on age, gender, activity level, and health state.

Sarcoidosis patients should consult with their doctors or certified dietitians to evaluate their individual nutritional needs. In general, a balanced diet with a range of nutrient-dense foods and suitable portion sizes is essential. This could include eating enough fruits and vegetables, integrating lean proteins into every meal, preferring whole grains over processed grains, and limiting your intake of added sweets and bad fats.

Nutrient-dense foods contain a high concentration of nutrients per calorie. Including these foods in meals can help sarcoidosis patients satisfy their nutritional requirements without ingesting too many calories. Here are some nutrient-dense foods to include in your meals:

Leafy greens such as spinach, kale, and Swiss chard.

Berries include blueberries, strawberries, and raspberries.

Fatty fish, including salmon, mackerel, and sardines.

Nuts and seeds include almonds, walnuts, chia seeds, and flaxseeds.

Legumes, including lentils, chickpeas, black beans, and kidney beans.

Whole grains include quinoa, brown rice, oats, and barley.

Colourful fruits and vegetables, like bell peppers, carrots, sweet potatoes, and tomatoes.

By including these nutrient-dense foods in your meals, you can optimize your nutrient intake and improve your overall health and well-being while managing sarcoidosis.

Low-Carb Lifestyle for Sarcoidosis Management

Sarcoidosis is a disorder in which granulomas, or microscopic clusters of inflammatory cells, grow in numerous organs of the body, most notably the lungs and lymph nodes. Sarcoidosis management requires a multifaceted strategy that includes medication, lifestyle modifications, and nutritional changes. One such dietary approach that is gaining popularity is low-carb living.

Low-carb eating for sarcoidosis control entails limiting carbohydrate intake, particularly refined carbs like as sweets and white flour, and prioritizing nutrient-dense, natural foods. Individuals with sarcoidosis may benefit from reducing their carbohydrate intake.

Advantages of a Low-Carb Approach in Managing Sarcoidosis Symptoms.

Taking a low-carb approach to controlling sarcoidosis symptoms can provide various advantages:

Reduced carbohydrate intake stabilizes blood sugar levels, aiding in managing sarcoidosis symptoms including fatigue and energy fluctuations.

Low-carb diets can help manage weight, which is crucial for people with sarcoidosis.

Excess weight can worsen symptoms and strain the body.

Reduced Inflammation: Refined carbs can lead to inflammation in the body. Individuals who limit their intake may experience less inflammation, which can help alleviate sarcoidosis symptoms.

Low-carb diets can improve energy levels and help manage fatigue associated with sarcoidosis.

Understanding Carbohydrates and their Effects on Blood Sugar

Carbohydrates are macronutrients found in many foods, such as grains, fruits, vegetables, and dairy products. When carbs are ingested, they are converted into glucose, which enters the bloodstream and boosts blood sugar levels. Blood sugar changes can worsen symptoms and have an influence on the overall health of people with sarcoidosis.

Carbohydrates have different impacts on blood sugar. Simple carbs, including sugars and refined grains, break down fast and can produce sudden blood sugar rises. Complex carbs, such as whole grains, legumes, and vegetables, are absorbed more slowly, leading to more stable blood sugar levels.

Individuals with sarcoidosis can improve blood sugar control and reduce the likelihood of symptom flare-ups by eating carbohydrates with a lower glycemic index (GI) and focusing on full, unprocessed meals.

CHAPTER THREE

Making low-carb substitutions for high-carb favorites is an important part of implementing a low-carb lifestyle for sarcoidosis treatment. Below are some examples of low-carb swaps:

Use cauliflower rice or zucchini noodles instead of standard rice or pasta to cut carbs while still enjoying familiar foods.

Use lettuce leaves instead of tortillas or bread for wraps or sandwiches to reduce carbs and enhance vegetable intake.

Use almond or coconut flour instead of wheat flour to make low-carb bread, muffins, and pancakes.

Instead of pasta, use spaghetti squash as a base for meals like spaghetti and meatballs or pasta primavera.

Sample low-carb meal plans and recipes.

Creating a sample low-carb meal plan can assist sarcoidosis patients manage their dietary choices and ensure they are obtaining the nutrients they require while limiting carbohydrate intake. Below is an example of a day's worth of low-carb meals:

Breakfast: Spinach and feta omelet, served with avocado slices.

Lunch option: Grilled chicken Caesar salad with romaine lettuce, grilled chicken breast, Parmesan cheese, and homemade dressing.

Dinner was baked fish, roasted asparagus, and cauliflower mashed potatoes.

Snacks include almonds, celery sticks with almond butter, and cherry tomatoes with mozzarella cheese.

Tips to Maintain a Low-Carb Lifestyle

Living a low-carb lifestyle needs dedication and planning. Here are some pointers for success:

Plan meals and snacks ahead of time to maximize nutrient density and reduce carbohydrate intake.

Read food labels to discover hidden carbohydrate sources such as added sugars and starches.

Eat complete, unprocessed foods including fruits, vegetables, lean meats, and healthy fats.

Stay Hydrated: Drinking enough water throughout the day promotes general health.

Adjust your diet based on your body's reactions to different foods to properly control symptoms.

Individuals with sarcoidosis who follow these suggestions and include low-carb living into their daily routine can improve their health and well-being while better controlling their symptoms.

Sarcoidosis Relief Recipes with High Antioxidant Content

Sarcoidosis is a disorder marked by the formation of small collections of inflammatory cells in many regions of the body, most notably the lungs and lymph nodes. While the specific etiology is uncertain, inflammation is a crucial factor in its advancement. Antioxidants, which are found in many foods, are powerful molecules that fight inflammation by neutralizing damaging free radicals in the body. Incorporating antioxidant-rich meals into your diet can help treat sarcoidosis symptoms while also promoting overall health.

Investigating the Potential of Antioxidants in Fighting Inflammation

Antioxidants are substances that prevent oxidation, a chemical reaction that can generate free radicals and trigger chain reactions that can harm cells. Inflammation, a critical component of sarcoidosis, is the body's immunological response to damaging stimuli. However, prolonged inflammation can cause tissue damage and aggravate sarcoidosis symptoms. Antioxidants counteract this process by scavenging free radicals, which reduces inflammation and prevents oxidative damage.

According to research, eating antioxidant-rich foods may help reduce the inflammation linked with sarcoidosis. Foods rich in vitamins C and E, beta-carotene, selenium, and flavonoids are very efficient at combating oxidative stress. These nutrients can be found in fruits, vegetables, nuts, seeds, and some spices. By having a mix of these foods in your diet, you can use antioxidants to help your body's natural defense systems against inflammation.

Superfoods: Their Antioxidant Properties

Superfoods are nutrient-dense foods that provide numerous health advantages, including antioxidants. Incorporating superfoods into your diet can give you with an abundance of vitamins, minerals, and antioxidants, all of which support overall health and wellness. Antioxidant-rich superfoods include berries (blueberries, strawberries, and raspberries), leafy greens (kale, spinach, and Swiss chard), nuts and seeds (almonds, walnuts, and chia seeds), and colorful vegetables (bell peppers, carrots, and tomatoes).

These superfoods contain high levels of antioxidants, such as vitamins C and E, beta-carotene, and flavonoids, which can protect cells from free radical damage and reduce inflammation. By including a range of superfoods in your diet, you can increase your antioxidant intake while also supporting your body's ability to manage sarcoidosis-related inflammation.

Delicious antioxidant-rich recipes for breakfast, lunch, and dinner.

Creating delicious and nutritious meals high in antioxidants is critical for managing sarcoidosis and improving overall health. Breakfast, lunch, and dinner are all opportunities to include antioxidant-rich products in your meals in unique and enjoyable ways.

For breakfast, try a berry smoothie with spinach, kale, blueberries, and almond milk. For lunch, try a colorful salad with mixed greens, bell peppers, tomatoes, carrots, avocado, and walnuts, topped with a homemade vinaigrette made from olive oil and balsamic vinegar. For dinner, try grilled salmon with roasted sweet potatoes and asparagus, seasoned with herbs and spices such as turmeric and ginger.

These recipes not only give a pleasant and delicious dining experience, but they also include a high concentration of antioxidants that help reduce inflammation and promote general health.

Snack Ideas Packed With Antioxidants

Snacking is a good opportunity to increase your antioxidant consumption throughout the day. Instead of grabbing processed snacks high in sugar and bad fats, choose nutritional foods rich in antioxidants to support your health and well-being.

Fresh fruit, such as berries, apples, and grapes, can be combined with nuts or seeds to provide additional protein and healthy fats. Vegetable sticks like carrots, cucumbers, and bell peppers can be paired with hummus or guacamole for a tasty and nutritious snack. Additionally, homemade trail mix made from a variety of nuts, seeds, and dried fruits is a practical and portable way to nourish your body with antioxidants while on the road.

By eating antioxidant-rich snacks, you can help your body's natural anti-inflammatory mechanisms and improve overall health and wellness.

Incorporating Antioxidant Drinks into Your Daily Routine

Beverages, like food, can include antioxidants to help you maintain your health and well-being. Incorporating antioxidant-rich beverages into your daily routine is a simple yet efficient approach to increasing your consumption of these beneficial substances.

Green tea is one of the most popular antioxidant-rich beverages, with high levels of catechins, which have been found to lower inflammation and protect against chronic diseases. Drinking green tea in the morning or throughout the day can provide numerous health benefits. Other antioxidant-rich beverages include freshly brewed coffee, which includes chlorogenic acid and other polyphenols, as well as fruit and vegetable juices produced from berries, spinach, and kale.

By integrating antioxidant-rich beverages into your daily routine, you can help your body's natural defense mechanisms against inflammation while also promoting overall health and wellness.

CHAPTER FOUR

Anti-inflammatory Cooking Techniques

Incorporating anti-inflammatory cooking techniques into your culinary repertoire will help you manage sarcoidosis and improve your health. Anti-inflammatory cooking focuses on products and practices that reduce inflammation in the body, which is critical for people with sarcoidosis.

One of the most basic principles in anti-inflammatory cooking is to prioritize whole, unprocessed foods. These foods, like fruits, vegetables, healthy grains, and lean proteins, are high in nutrients and antioxidants that help fight inflammation. Including these items in your meals is the foundation of an anti-inflammatory diet.

Furthermore, cooking methods are important in maintaining foods' anti-inflammatory qualities. Steaming, sautéing, and baking instead of frying can help keep items nutritionally intact. These milder procedures reduce the development of toxic chemicals, which can increase inflammation.

Furthermore, emphasizing variation and color in your meals is essential. Aim to include a range of colorful fruits and vegetables in your meals, as different colors frequently indicate distinct nutritional profiles. For example, the brilliant tints seen in fruits like berries and veggies like spinach signal the presence of powerful antioxidants that fight inflammation and support general health.

Finally, adding plant-based protein sources like legumes, nuts, and seeds can be useful. These meals are high in protein, but they also include phytonutrients and fiber, which have anti-inflammatory qualities. By including these items in your meals, you can improve their nutritional content while also helping to manage sarcoidosis-related inflammation.

In summary, anti-inflammatory cooking approaches focus on complete, nutrient-dense foods, use mild cooking methods, embrace culinary diversity, and use plant-based proteins. Individuals with sarcoidosis can improve their general health and well-being by incorporating these strategies into their diets.

Understanding Inflammation's Role in Sarcoidosis

To effectively manage sarcoidosis with dietary changes, it is critical to understand the role of inflammation in the disease. Sarcoidosis is distinguished by the presence of granulomas—small aggregates of inflammatory cells—in several organs, most notably the lungs and lymph nodes.

These granulomas can disrupt organ function, resulting in symptoms such as coughing, shortness of breath, and exhaustion.

Inflammation is the body's normal immunological response to adverse stimuli like infections or tissue damage. However, in disorders such as sarcoidosis, the immune system is dysregulated, resulting in chronic inflammation and the production of granulomas.

Dietary choices can alter the body's inflammatory processes. Certain foods, such as processed meats, refined sugars, and trans fats, might increase inflammation and worsen sarcoidosis symptoms. On the other hand, eating an anti-inflammatory diet high in fruits, vegetables, whole grains, and healthy fats can help reduce inflammation and improve overall health.

Sarcoidosis inflammation is complex, including a wide range of immune cells, cytokines, and signaling pathways. Dietary changes may not cure the problem on their own, but they can help to reduce inflammation and improve general health.

Individuals can support their health goals by understanding the inflammatory mechanisms involved in sarcoidosis, as well as the importance of nutrition in controlling inflammation.

Consulting with healthcare professionals, such as registered dietitians or healthcare providers who specialize in sarcoidosis management, can provide personalized advice on dietary strategies adapted to individual needs.

Cooking Methods for Preserving Anti-Inflammatory Properties in Foods

Preserving foods' anti-inflammatory qualities while cooking is critical for maximizing their health benefits, particularly for those with sarcoidosis. Certain cooking procedures can help to preserve nutrients and antioxidants while reducing the development of toxic chemicals that can cause inflammation.

Steaming is a mild cooking method that preserves the nutritional value of foods, especially vegetables. Cooking vegetables with steam preserves their vitamins, minerals, and phytonutrients, which contribute to their anti-inflammatory qualities. Steaming veggies also helps them retain their brilliant colors and crisp texture, which improves both their visual appeal and nutritional value.

Sautéing is another approach for preserving foods' anti-inflammatory benefits. When sautéing, choose healthy fats like olive or avocado oil, which include monounsaturated fats and antioxidants that help fight inflammation. Furthermore, sautéing allows you to swiftly cook veggies over high heat, conserving their nutrients while imparting flavor.

Baking is a versatile cooking technique that may be used to create a variety of anti-inflammatory foods. When baking items like fish or poultry, use herbs, spices, and citrus zest to add flavor without relying on too much salt or bad fats. Baking also helps you to cook items evenly without using extra oils, making it a healthier alternative to frying.

Including raw foods in your meals, such as salads or crudité platters, can provide a refreshing and nutrient-dense boost to your diet. Raw fruits and vegetables are high in enzymes, vitamins, and antioxidants, which promote the body's anti-inflammatory pathways. To reduce pesticide and other pollutant exposure, properly wash fresh vegetables and opt for organic products whenever possible.

Individuals with sarcoidosis can optimize their dietary choices by incorporating cooking methods that preserve foods' anti-inflammatory qualities. Experimenting with different techniques and recipes can provide variety and excitement to your meals while also increasing their nutritional worth.

CHAPTER FIVE

Meal preparation is an important part of treating sarcoidosis through nutrition, especially for people with busy lifestyles. The aim is to streamline the process so that healthy eating becomes both convenient and

Set aside time each week to plan your meals. When developing your strategy, take into account your schedule, dietary limitations, and nutritional requirements.

Prepare large batches of staple foods such as grains, proteins, and veggies ahead of time. This helps you to prepare quick and healthy meals all week.

Invest in kitchen gadgets such as slow cookers, pressure cookers, or rice cookers to save time during cooking. These appliances allow you to cook enormous amounts of food with minimal effort.

Prepare ingredients for the week by washing, cutting, and portioning them ahead of time. This saves time while preparing meals and encourages you to choose healthier options when you're hungry.

Maintain portion control by packaging meals in individual containers or portion sizes for easy grab-and-go throughout the week. This avoids overeating and helps you stay to your nutritional goals.

Importance of Meal Preparation in Sarcoidosis Management:

Meal preparation is essential for treating sarcoidosis since it promotes a balanced diet and lifestyle. Here's why it matters:

Maintaining a balanced diet is crucial for treating sarcoidosis symptoms and improving overall health. Meal planning ensures that healthy selections are easily accessible, limiting the temptation to choose convenience meals that may exacerbate symptoms.

To manage sarcoidosis, a healthy diet can help decrease inflammation and boost immunological function. Meal preparation allows you to include a range of nutrient-dense foods in your meals, such as fruits, vegetables, lean proteins, and whole grains, encouraging overall nutrition.

Time Efficiency: Sarcoidosis patients may struggle to cook daily meals due to exhaustion and other symptoms. Meal preparation saves time and energy by front-loading the cooking process, making it easier to maintain a nutritious diet even on hectic days.

Proper portion management helps manage weight and prevent sarcoidosis problems. Pre-portioning meals during meal prep allows you to consume suitable serving amounts while avoiding overeating.

Meal prep allows for customized meals based on your nutritional needs and tastes. Whether you follow a certain diet or have food allergies, prepping meals ahead of time provides you more control over your eating habits.

Tips for Effective Meal Planning and Preparation:

Efficient meal planning and preparation are critical for success while treating sarcoidosis through nutrition. Here are some ideas to simplify the process:

Make a Master Grocery List: Before shopping, make a list of all the ingredients you'll need for your meals. To save time while shopping, organize the list by food category.

Choose versatile foods to reduce waste and simplify meal preparation. Roasted veggies, for example, can be used all week in salads, grain bowls, and wraps.

Schedule weekly food prep sessions. Set aside a few hours on the weekend or a less stressful day to cut vegetables, cook grains, and prepare proteins in advance.

Prepare freezer-friendly recipes for future use. Soups, stews, and casseroles typically store well and may be reheated for quick and easy dinners.

Invest in reusable storage containers of various sizes to accommodate meal quantities. Choose containers that are microwave-safe, dishwasher-safe, and stackable for convenient storage.

Stay Flexible: Planning is important, but it's also important to adjust to changes in schedule and preferences. Keep a variety of quick and easy dinner options on hand for days when meal planning is not possible.

Batch cooking is a time-saving meal preparation strategy that entails making big amounts of food at once to be consumed throughout the week. Here are some batch-cooking methods to consider:

Create hearty one-pot meals like chili, curry, or stir-fries with a range of ingredients and flavors. These meals are not only easy to prepare but also require minimal cleaning.

Bulk cook grains like rice, quinoa, or pasta for numerous meals. Cooked grains can be stored in the refrigerator or freezer for rapid meal assembling.

By roasting veggies in bulk, you may enhance the flavor and nutrition of your meals. Cut up a variety of vegetables, mix with olive oil and seasonings, then roast on a large sheet pan until soft. Roasted vegetables can be used throughout the week in salads, wraps, and grain bowls.

Protein Prep: Cook a large quantity of protein sources like chicken breasts, tofu, or legumes to use in various meals. Season proteins with herbs and spices to increase flavor variety.

Freeze meal components such as sauces, marinades, and cooked meats in individual amounts. These can be easily thawed and blended with fresh ingredients for simple meal preparation.

Storage and reheating instructions for prepared meals:

Proper storage and reheating are critical to preserving the quality and safety of cooked meals. Here are a few guidelines to follow:

Refrigerate cooked meals in sealed containers for up to 3-4 days. To prevent bacterial growth, keep the refrigerator temperature at or below 40°F (4°C).

For long-term storage, freeze prepared meals in freezer-safe containers or resealable bags. Label containers with the date and contents to facilitate identification. Most frozen meals can be kept for up to three months.

To maintain food safety, reheat prepared meals in a microwave, hob, or oven until they reach 165°F (74°C). Stir or rotate the meal halfway through the cooking phase to achieve even heating.

Avoid reheating some dishes, such as shellfish and dairy-based sauces, as they may develop an undesirable texture or flavor. To keep meals fresh, consider adding these items just before serving.

CHAPTER SIX

Creating Personalised Meal Plans for Your Lifestyle:

Creating personalized meal planning based on your lifestyle is critical for long-term success in treating sarcoidosis through nutrition. Here's how to make a personalized meal plan.

Consider dietary limitations, allergies, and intolerances when creating a meal plan. For personalized suggestions, see a healthcare physician or a qualified dietitian.

Incorporate favorite foods and flavors into your meal plan for maximum enjoyment and satisfaction. Experiment with new recipes and ingredients to keep meals interesting and diverse.

Balance Macronutrients: Eat a variety of carbohydrates, proteins, and fats to maintain energy and satiety. Choose entire dietary sources of macronutrients such as lean proteins, whole grains, and good fats.

Plan for Variety: Include a variety of fruits, vegetables, grains, and proteins in your meal plan to acquire a wide range of nutrients. Rotate your meal alternatives throughout the week to avoid boredom and guarantee proper nourishment.

Plan meals around your schedule and tastes. Aim for regular, balanced meals spread out throughout the day to maintain steady energy levels and promote overall health.

Be Flexible: A meal plan can provide structure, but it's important to be adaptable to changes in schedule and appetites. Allow for occasional indulgences like dining out while maintaining portion control and overall nutritional balance.

By applying these tactics, you can effectively manage sarcoidosis through nutrition while taking into account your hectic schedule and personal preferences. Consistent meal preparation, deliberate planning, and customization are essential for long-term success in living a healthy lifestyle.

Managing Symptoms with Flavoured Soups and Salads

Sarcoidosis, a disorder that causes inflammation in numerous organs of the body, frequently necessitates cautious symptom treatment. While medicine is important for treatment, food choices can also have a substantial impact on symptom management. Flavorful soups and salads can be useful additions to a diet for treating sarcoidosis symptoms.

Soups and salads have various health benefits for people with sarcoidosis. They make it simple to add a range of nutrient-dense items to your meals, such as veggies, lean proteins, and healthy fats. Furthermore, the high water content in soups and the fiber in salads can aid in hydration and digestive health, both of which are necessary for overall well-being.

Including soups and salads in a sarcoidosis control diet has various benefits. For starters, these foods are often high in vitamins, minerals, and antioxidants, which can boost the immune system and reduce inflammation. For example, plants such as spinach, kale, and bell peppers are high in vitamins A, C, and K, as well as phytochemicals having anti-inflammatory qualities.

Furthermore, soups and salads are adaptable and can be tailored to certain dietary constraints and preferences. They offer a wonderful opportunity to experiment with various flavors and textures while maintaining a well-balanced dinner. Individuals can improve their overall health by eating a variety of nutrients.

Nutritious Soup Recipes for Healing and Comfort

When developing soup recipes for sarcoidosis management, it is critical to prioritize nutrient density and flavor. Incorporating legumes, whole grains, and lean proteins into soups can boost their nutritional content while also delivering sustained energy and inducing satiety. For example, lentil soup with tomatoes and kale is not only a hearty and satisfying dinner, but it also contains a lot of minerals like fiber, iron, and vitamin K.

Incorporating anti-inflammatory herbs and spices like turmeric, ginger, and garlic can also improve the therapeutic benefits of soups. These components not only offer a depth of flavor but also help to reduce inflammation and boost immunological function. Experimenting with different combinations of veggies, herbs, and spices can help people develop soup recipes that meet their cravings while also supporting their health goals.

Creative Salad Ideas with a Nutritional Punch

Salads are another wonderful option for sarcoidosis patients, providing a refreshing and nutrient-dense meal. To boost the nutritional value of salads, add a range of colorful vegetables, leafy greens, and protein-rich toppings.

A Mediterranean-inspired salad, for example, that includes mixed greens, cherry tomatoes, cucumbers, olives, feta cheese, and grilled chicken, is a great mixture of flavors and nutrients.

Salads can be made even more anti-inflammatory by including omega-3 fatty acid-rich items like walnuts, flaxseeds, and salmon. These good fats not only improve heart health but also assist in controlling the immunological response and minimizing sarcoidosis-related inflammation. Adding a tasty vinaigrette made with olive oil, lemon juice, and herbs helps bring the salad together while also delivering health benefits.

Adding Protein and Healthy Fats to Soups and Salads.

Protein and healthy fats are crucial components of a sarcoidosis treatment diet because they include nutrients required for tissue repair and immunological function. When making soups and salads, make sure to incorporate lean protein sources such as chicken, turkey, fish, tofu, and lentils. These protein-rich foods help to preserve muscle mass, boost energy levels, and increase satiety.

Similarly, adding healthy fats to soups and salads can increase their nutritional worth. Avocados, nuts, seeds, and olive oil are high in monounsaturated fats, which have been demonstrated to reduce inflammation and improve heart health. Including these items not only adds creaminess and richness to soups and salads but also improves nutrient absorption and promotes overall health.

Tips for enhancing flavor without sacrificing nutrition

While flavor is important for enjoying meals, soups and salads can be made more tasty without sacrificing nutritious value. One method is to utilize herbs, spices, and citrus zest to enhance the depth and complexity of recipes. Fresh herbs such as basil, cilantro, and parsley can improve the flavor of soups and salads while also adding antioxidants and minerals.

Roasting or grilling veggies before incorporating them into soups and salads can help enhance their flavor and produce a delectable smokiness. Similarly, using umami-rich items like mushrooms, soy sauce, or miso paste can improve the savory notes of recipes without relying on too much salt or fat. Experimenting with different flavor combinations and cooking methods can assist folks in creating pleasant and healthy soups and salads that support their sarcoidosis management goals.

Hearty and Nutritious Main Courses: Sarcoidosis is a disorder that frequently requires dietary changes to adequately control symptoms. Main courses have an

important function in giving nutrition while
also making meals satisfying and
pleasurable.

CHAPTER SEVEN

Protein and fiber are essential components of a diet designed to effectively treat sarcoidosis. Protein aids in tissue repair and regeneration strengthens the immune system, and promotes overall health. It is especially important for people with sarcoidosis because it promotes muscular strength and healing, especially during times of inflammation. Lean proteins, such as poultry, fish, and lentils, are ideal choices since they supply critical nutrients without adding unnecessary fat.

Fibre, on the other hand, is necessary for digestive health and can help manage symptoms like constipation, which is prevalent with sarcoidosis. Whole grains, fruits, vegetables, and legumes are high-fiber foods that should be consumed regularly.

A Sarcoidosis Management Diet Cookbook should focus on recipes high in protein and fiber. These nutrients not only enhance overall health but also help sarcoidosis patients control symptoms and improve their quality of life.

Creating delicious and substantial main course recipes is critical for adhering to a Sarcoidosis Management Diet. Variety is important since it keeps meals interesting and pleasurable. Recipes should incorporate a variety of lean proteins, nutritious grains, and veggies to provide nutritional needs while satisfying hunger.

For example, grilled chicken with quinoa and roasted veggies or lentil curry with brown rice has protein, fiber, and complex carbohydrates that help keep you full and content.

Incorporating herbs, spices, and tasty sauces can improve the taste of dishes without using too much salt or fat, making them safe for people with sarcoidosis.

Individuals with sarcoidosis can benefit from a broad and healthy diet that includes a variety of lean proteins and plant-based alternatives, as outlined in the cookbook.

Delicious Side Dishes to Complement Main Courses:

While main courses take the stage, side dishes are essential for rounding out meals and adding extra nutrients and flavors. Satisfying side dishes should complement the main course and provide a diversity of textures and flavors.

Sarcoidosis patients should eat nutrient-dense side dishes such as steamed vegetables, salads, and whole grains. These foods are rich in vitamins, minerals, and fiber, and they help you feel full and satisfied.

The Sarcoidosis Management Diet Cookbook includes a range of side dishes, allowing users to make balanced meals that fit their nutritional needs and taste preferences.

Portion control and balance for optimum nutrition:

Individuals with sarcoidosis must maintain proper portion management to manage their weight and nutrition. While it is vital to include a range of nutrient-dense meals in one's diet, doing so in proper portions helps to prevent overeating and improves digestion.

Recipes in the Sarcoidosis Management Diet Cookbook should include portion size recommendations as well as ideas for balancing meals to guarantee the proper nutritional balance. Encouraging mindful eating behaviors, such as eating slowly and paying attention to hunger and fullness cues, can also assist sarcoidosis patients in maintaining a healthy weight and improving their overall health.

Individuals can learn how to make pleasant meals that meet their health objectives and efficiently manage their condition by focusing on portion control and balance in the cookbook.

Indulgent but healthy desserts and snacks: Managing sarcoidosis through nutrition typically necessitates balancing health concerns with a desire for rich foods. Fortunately, you may enjoy delectable desserts and snacks without sacrificing your nutritional goals. Indulgent yet healthy options focus on nutrient-dense components like fruits, nuts, and whole grains while limiting added sweets, processed flour, and bad fats. These delicacies can curb cravings while also improving general health and well-being.

A fruit and nut energy ball is a tempting but healthful dessert. These bite-sized sweets include dates, almonds, and seeds, with a hint of natural sweetness from honey or maple syrup. They're high in fiber, healthy fats, and antioxidants, making them an excellent choice for satisfying cravings without derailing your diet.

Satisfying Your Sweet Tooth While Maintaining Your Health:

Sarcoidosis care frequently includes making lifestyle modifications, including dietary changes, to promote optimal health. When it comes to gratifying your sugar desire, you need to look for options that are both tasty and nutritious.

This entails selecting foods that are low in added sugars, refined carbohydrates, and harmful fats while yet offering the satisfaction and enjoyment you seek.

Experimenting with natural sweeteners such as stevia, monk fruit, or raw honey can help you fulfill your sweet desire without jeopardizing your health. These alternatives can sweeten desserts and snacks without raising blood sugar levels or creating inflammation, which is especially essential for people with sarcoidosis. Combining sweets with nutrient-dense items such as fruits, nuts, and dark chocolate can result in satisfying snacks that promote general health and well-being.

Low-Carb Dessert Recipes That Will Not Increase Blood Sugar:

Maintaining stable blood sugar levels is critical for people with sarcoidosis in terms of symptom management and general health. Low-carb dessert dishes can be a useful addition to a sarcoidosis treatment diet because they help reduce blood sugar surges, which can increase inflammation and other symptoms of the condition.

Low-carb dessert recipes include almond flour cookies, avocado chocolate mousse, and coconut flour pancakes. These recipes employ different flours and sugars to cut carbs while still providing excellent flavors and textures. By including these desserts in your diet, you may enjoy sweet treats without worrying about how they affect your blood sugar levels.

Healthy Snack Options for Sarcoidosis Management:

Snacking is a key part of managing sarcoidosis because it provides energy and nutrients in between meals, which promotes overall health and wellness. Healthy snack ideas for sarcoidosis management include full, nutrient-dense meals that give sustained energy and encourage satiety while reducing inflammation and other symptoms of the condition.

Healthy snacks for managing sarcoidosis include Greek yogurt with berries, mixed nuts, and seeds, veggie sticks with hummus, and sliced apples with almond butter. These snacks are high in protein, fiber, and healthy fats, which assist in maintaining blood sugar levels and avoiding energy dumps throughout the day. By including these snacks in your diet plan, you can improve your general health while effectively treating sarcoidosis symptoms.

CHAPTER EIGHT

Mindful eating approaches can be useful tools for people with sarcoidosis who want to indulge in delights in moderation while still meeting their health goals. Mindful eating is focusing on the sensory experience of eating, such as the taste, texture, and aroma of food, as well as recognizing hunger and fullness cues to avoid overeating.

Mindful eating can help people with sarcoidosis eat foods in moderation by helping them savor each bite and completely appreciate the flavors without feeling restricted or guilty.

Techniques like eating slowly, chewing properly, and paying attention to hunger and fullness cues can help prevent overindulgence and foster a healthy relationship with food.

By incorporating mindful eating into your daily routine, you may enjoy sweets in moderation while also improving your overall health and well-being.

Incorporating desserts and snacks into your meal plan is a crucial part of managing sarcoidosis because it ensures that you obtain the nutrients you need to support your health and well-being while still enjoying your favorite foods.

When preparing meals, it's critical to evaluate the nutritional value of desserts and snacks, as well as how they fit into your overall dietary objectives.

One way to incorporate desserts and snacks into your meal plan is to pair them with nutrient-dense meals such as fruits, vegetables, whole grains, and lean protein.

This can assist ensure that you satisfy your dietary requirements while also allowing you indulgent delights in moderation. Furthermore, spacing out snacks and desserts throughout the day can help prevent energy dumps and keep blood sugar levels stable, promoting overall health and well-being. By taking a balanced approach to meal planning, you can eat a variety of foods while efficiently managing sarcoidosis symptoms and improving your overall health.

Lifestyle Tips for Long-Term Sarcoidosis Management.

Sarcoidosis is a complex disorder that affects several systems in the body, and treating it requires a holistic approach. Long-term management relies heavily on lifestyle adjustments, which aid in symptom reduction, overall health improvement, and improved quality of life.

Nutrition: A well-balanced diet helps boost immune function and minimize inflammation caused by sarcoidosis. Focus on full, nutrient-dense foods including fruits, vegetables, whole grains, lean meats, and healthy fats. Some people may find relief from their symptoms by avoiding certain trigger foods, such as processed foods, dairy, or gluten. Working with a licensed dietitian can help you personalize your food plan to your specific needs and interests.

Hydration: Staying hydrated is important for overall health and can help prevent sarcoidosis complications such as kidney stones. Drink plenty of water throughout the day and restrict your intake of sugary and caffeine-containing beverages.

Stress Management: Chronic stress can increase sarcoidosis symptoms and have a detrimental influence on overall health.

Incorporate stress-reduction techniques into your routine, such as mindfulness meditation, deep breathing exercises, yoga, or spending time outside. Finding activities that encourage relaxation and a sense of peace can assist in reducing stress and discomfort.

Sleep: Adequate sleep is essential for immunological function, energy levels, and general wellness. Aim for 7-9 hours of good sleep per night and create a peaceful bedtime ritual.

Make your sleeping environment as comfortable as possible, free of distractions like electronics and excessive noise. If you are experiencing sleep difficulties, consult a healthcare specialist for personalized recommendations and treatment choices.

Smoking cessation: Smoking can exacerbate sarcoidosis symptoms and raise the risk of consequences like lung damage. If you smoke, quitting is one of the most important things you can do to improve your health and manage your disease. Seek aid from healthcare professionals, smoking cessation programs, or support groups to successfully quit.

Regular Monitoring: Keep track of your symptoms, medications, and lifestyle habits to better understand how they affect your condition. Regular visits to healthcare experts can help monitor illness progression, change treatment plans as required, and address any concerns or issues that occur.

Individuals with sarcoidosis who follow these lifestyle guidelines can empower themselves to take an active role in managing their condition and enhancing their overall health and well-being.

Beyond Diet: Other Lifestyle Factors That Affect Sarcoidosis Symptoms

While diet is important for treating sarcoidosis symptoms, other lifestyle factors can also have an impact on the disease's progression and overall well-being. Addressing these characteristics, in addition to making dietary adjustments, can help people with sarcoidosis better manage their disease and enhance their quality of life.

Environmental Exposures: Pollution, allergies, and occupational dangers can increase sarcoidosis symptoms and cause flare-ups. When possible, limiting exposure to certain triggers can help alleviate symptom severity and improve respiratory function. This may entail utilizing air purifiers, avoiding known allergies, and exercising caution in work environments.

Sun Exposure: Some people with sarcoidosis may have photosensitivity, which means that exposure to sunlight can aggravate skin lesions or cause flare-ups. Wearing protective clothes, applying sunscreen, and seeking shade when outdoors can all help to reduce symptoms and prevent consequences.

Emotional Well-Being: The emotional toll of living with a chronic illness such as sarcoidosis should not be underestimated. Managing stress, anxiety, and depression is critical for general well-being and may aid in symptom reduction. Seeking help from friends, family, support groups, or mental health experts can help you develop coping methods and gain emotional support.

Medication Adherence: Effective sarcoidosis management requires adherence to recommended drugs and treatment programs. Skipping doses or quitting drugs without medical supervision might result in worsened symptoms and disease progression. Open communication with healthcare providers about any concerns or side effects can assist ensure that treatment strategies are tailored to each patient's specific requirements and preferences.

Healthy Relationships: Having healthy, supportive relationships with friends, family, and healthcare providers helps improve mental and emotional health. Surrounding oneself with a supporting network of people who understand and empathize with the difficulties of living with sarcoidosis can provide you inspiration, motivation, and a sense of belonging.

Pacing Activities: Balancing activity and rest is critical for maintaining energy levels and avoiding weariness, which is a typical symptom of sarcoidosis. Pace yourself throughout the day, prioritizing activities and taking breaks when necessary to save energy and avoid overexertion. Listening to your body and respecting its limits might help you avoid symptom exacerbation and enhance overall performance.

Individuals with sarcoidosis can improve their overall quality of life by addressing these lifestyle factors as well as nutritional adjustments.

CHAPTER NINE

Stress management and appropriate sleep are critical in the treatment of sarcoidosis, affecting both physical and mental well-being. Incorporating stress-reduction measures and improving sleep quality can assist people with sarcoidosis manage their symptoms and improve their overall quality of life.

Chronic stress can worsen the inflammation and immunological dysfunction associated with sarcoidosis, resulting in increased symptom severity and disease progression. Stress can also cause fatigue, anxiety, depression, and other emotional symptoms that are frequent among people suffering from chronic illnesses. Individuals with sarcoidosis can enhance their overall health by appropriately managing stress.

Stress Management approaches: People with sarcoidosis can use a variety of stress management approaches in their daily lives to improve relaxation and reduce stress levels. These could include mindfulness meditation, deep breathing exercises, gradual muscular relaxation, yoga, tai chi, or guided visualization. Finding activities that generate a sense of peace and well-being can help people cope with the challenges of living with sarcoidosis while also improving their overall quality of life.

Importance of Sleep: Adequate sleep is critical for immunological function, energy, cognitive function, and overall health. Individuals with sarcoidosis frequently experience sleep problems, which can increase symptoms such as exhaustion, discomfort, and cognitive failure. Individuals with sarcoidosis can improve their sleep quality and overall well-being by prioritizing sleep and implementing healthy sleep habits such as sticking to a regular sleep schedule, developing a calming bedtime routine, and creating a pleasant sleep environment.

Sleep Hygiene Tips: Practicing excellent sleep hygiene can assist sarcoidosis patients to improve their sleep quality and prevent sleep disruptions.

This may involve avoiding stimulants like caffeine and nicotine close to bedtime, limiting screen time before bed, providing a quiet and distraction-free sleep environment, and indulging in soothing activities like reading or taking a warm bath. If sleep difficulties persist despite these precautions, people should consult with their doctor for additional diagnosis and treatment.

(CBT-I): Cognitive-behavioral therapy for insomnia (CBT-I) is a highly effective, evidence-based treatment for sleep difficulties that sarcoidosis patients frequently suffer. CBT-I enables people to identify and address maladaptive beliefs and behaviors that contribute to insomnia, supporting healthier sleep patterns and enhancing overall sleep quality. Individuals with sarcoidosis who have chronic sleep difficulties may benefit from CBT-I, either alone or in conjunction with other treatments.

Individuals with sarcoidosis can improve their general well-being and capacity to manage their symptoms by focusing on stress management and getting enough sleep.

Safely incorporating physical activity into your routine.

Physical activity is essential for sarcoidosis management since it improves cardiovascular health, muscle strength, flexibility, and general well-being. Individuals with sarcoidosis, on the other hand, must approach exercise with caution and consideration for their specific symptoms and limits.

Benefits of Exercise: Regular exercise has various advantages for people with sarcoidosis, including improved cardiovascular health, improved pulmonary function, increased muscle strength and endurance, improved mood, and reduced fatigue. Exercise can also help people maintain a healthy weight, reduce stress, and enhance their general quality of life.

Types of activity: People with sarcoidosis can incorporate a variety of exercises into their daily regimen, including aerobic activity, weight training, flexibility exercises, and balance exercises.

Aerobic exercise, such as walking, cycling, swimming, or dancing, enhances cardiovascular fitness and endurance. Strength training exercises, such as lifting weights or utilizing resistance bands, aid in muscle strength development and prevent muscle atrophy.

Yoga and stretching are two flexibility activities that can help you enhance your range of motion. Tai chi and standing on one leg are examples of balancing exercises that can help increase stability.

Exercise Guidelines: Before beginning or modifying an exercise program, individuals with sarcoidosis should check with their healthcare professional to confirm that the chosen activities are safe and appropriate for their specific needs and abilities.

Individuals should begin cautiously and progressively increase the intensity and duration of their workouts over time, paying attention to their bodies and avoiding activities that worsen symptoms or create discomfort. It's also critical to stay hydrated, warm up before exercising, and cool down afterward to avoid injury.

Pacing Activities: People with sarcoidosis should exercise slowly and avoid overexertion, especially if they are tired or have difficulty breathing. Breaking up exercise into shorter, more manageable bouts throughout the day can help to avoid exhaustion and maximize energy levels. It's also critical to prioritize rest and recovery, giving your body time to heal in between sessions.

Listen to Your Body: People with sarcoidosis should listen to their bodies and be aware of any warning signs or symptoms while exercising. If symptoms such as chest pain, dizziness, shortness of breath, or acute weariness appear, individuals should discontinue exercise immediately and seek medical attention if necessary. Adjusting the intensity or type of exercise as needed will help you avoid injury and have a safe and pleasurable workout.

Individuals with sarcoidosis can enhance their general health and well-being while also better managing their symptoms over time by introducing physical activity into their routine safely and gradually.

CHAPTER TEN

Living with sarcoidosis can be difficult, both physically and emotionally, but there are tools and support available to help people manage their condition successfully and enhance their quality of life. Seeking help from healthcare specialists and support groups can provide essential knowledge, encouragement, and emotional support as you journey through sarcoidosis.

Healthcare Team: Effective sarcoidosis management requires the formation of a supportive healthcare team. This could include primary care physicians, pulmonologists, rheumatologists, dermatologists, ophthalmologists, and other specialists who can provide complete care and support tailored to individual requirements.

Open communication with healthcare practitioners, asking questions, and advocating for one's needs are all essential components of self-care and empowerment.

Joining a support group for sarcoidosis patients can provide a sense of belonging, understanding, and validation. Support groups provide a secure environment in which to share experiences, ask questions, and trade practical advice and coping strategies for dealing with the challenges of living with sarcoidosis. Many support groups also offer educational resources, guest lecturers, and social gatherings to encourage relationships and mutual support.

Educational Resources: Knowing as much as possible about sarcoidosis, its symptoms, therapies, and management strategies can help people take an active role in their care.

Staying up to date on the latest research and breakthroughs in sarcoidosis therapy can also help patients make educated decisions regarding their care.

Sarcoidosis patient advocacy organizations provide advocacy, education, and support to those impacted by the condition. These organizations provide a variety of resources and services, such as educational materials, support groups, patient assistance programs, research funding, and advocacy campaigns targeted at increasing awareness and improving access to care for those living with sarcoidosis.

Individuals with sarcoidosis can obtain the information, encouragement, and emotional support they require to effectively manage their condition and improve their quality of life by seeking assistance and resources from healthcare providers, support groups, online communities, and patient advocacy organizations.

Maintaining Motivation and Commitment to Your Health Journey.

Living with a chronic condition like sarcoidosis necessitates a continuous commitment and determination to manage symptoms, stick to treatment plans, and prioritize self-care. While the trip may be difficult, remaining motivated and committed to one's health is critical for attaining the best results and keeping a great quality of life.

Setting Realistic Goals: Having realistic, attainable goals might assist sarcoidosis patients in staying motivated and focused on their health path. Break down huge goals into smaller, more doable tasks, and celebrate your accomplishments along the way. Setting precise, quantifiable objectives, whether they are for increasing exercise tolerance, adopting healthier eating habits, or managing stress more efficiently, can provide a sense of success and inspiration to keep going.

Finding Meaning and Purpose: Connecting with one's values, interests, and sources of meaning and purpose can help provide direction and motivation during challenging times. Participating in activities that bring joy, fulfillment, and a feeling of purpose can help people keep a positive attitude and resilience in the face of adversity. Finding meaning and purpose, whether via spending time with loved ones, pursuing hobbies, volunteering, or donating to worthwhile causes, can help people with sarcoidosis cope with the ups and downs of living with a chronic illness.

Cultivating Self-Compassion: Living with a chronic illness, such as sarcoidosis, can be difficult, and individuals must practice self-compassion and self-care throughout the process.

Be gentle to yourself, and recognize the courage, fortitude, and perseverance required to handle a chronic condition daily. Treat yourself with the same care, understanding, and empathy that you would show a friend facing comparable circumstances. Individuals can recharge and refill their energy levels by engaging in self-care activities such as relaxation techniques, hobbies, and spending time outside.

Seeking Support: Creating a strong support network of friends, family, healthcare providers, and peers can provide vital encouragement, direction, and emotional support as you navigate your sarcoidosis journey. When in need, seek assistance from others, and do not be afraid to ask for help or support when faced with a struggle. Joining support groups, going to educational events, and interacting with others who have had similar experiences can all help you feel more connected and validated.

Fostering Resilience: Developing resilience, or the ability to adapt and recover in the face of adversity, is critical for dealing with the difficulties of living with sarcoidosis. Concentrate on your strengths, coping abilities, and resources that have guided you through difficult circumstances in the past. Mindfulness, gratitude, and positive thinking can help you retain a resilient mindset and perspective. Remember that setbacks and problems are a normal part of the road, and each one you conquer makes you stronger and more resilient in the long run.

Individuals with sarcoidosis can empower themselves to manage their illness and live their best lives by remaining motivated, determined, and resilient in the face of obstacles. Celebrate your accomplishments, practice self-compassion, and rely on your support network for motivation and assistance along the road. With commitment, perseverance, and support, you may overcome barriers and thrive despite the difficulties of living with sarcoidosis.

Recipes:

Turmeric Lentil Soup: Turmeric is recognized for its anti-inflammatory effects, which may help people with sarcoidosis.

Salmon with Lemon-Dill Sauce: High in omega-3 fatty acids, salmon reduces inflammation and promotes overall heart health.

Quinoa and Roasted Vegetable Salad: Quinoa has protein and fiber, while roasted veggies include vitamins and minerals, making this a nutrient-dense meal.

Chickpea and Spinach Curry: Chickpeas are high in protein and fiber, and spinach provides iron and other critical elements.

Grilled Chicken Caesar Salad: The combination of lean chicken protein, lush greens, and a light dressing makes for a tasty and nutritious lunch.

Stuffed Bell Peppers with Turkey and Brown Rice: Bell peppers are high in antioxidants, while turkey and brown rice contain protein and fiber.

Mango Avocado Salsa with Baked Tortilla Chips: A delicious and nutritious snack.

Eggplant & Tomato Ratatouille: Eggplant is high in antioxidants and fiber, so this recipe is both tasty and nutritious.

Sweet Potato and Black Bean Tacos: Sweet potatoes are strong in beta-carotene, and black beans provide protein and fiber for a satisfying lunch.

Berry Smoothie with Spinach and Flaxseeds: A tasty and nutritious way to start the day, loaded with antioxidants, vitamins, and omega-3 fatty acids.

30 Day Meal Plan:

Week 1:

Day 1:

Breakfast: Berry smoothie with spinach and flaxseed.

Snack: Greek yogurt with honey.

Lunch: Turmeric lentil soup.

Snack: Carrot Sticks and Hummus.

Dinner: Grilled chicken Caesar salad.

Day 2:

Breakfast: Mango Avocado Smoothie Bowl.

Snack: almonds.

Lunch: Stuffed bell peppers with turkey and brown rice.

Snack: Apple slices and almond butter.

Dinner: Chickpea and Spinach Curry with Quinoa.

Continue to eat a variety of meals throughout the week, ensuring a healthy balance of lean proteins, fats, and complex carbohydrates.

Week 2:

Day 8:

Breakfast: Scrambled eggs with spinach and tomato.

Snack: Cottage Cheese and Pineapple.

Lunch: Salmon with Lemon-Dill Sauce and roasted vegetables.

Snack: Mixed berries.

Dinner: Sweet potato and black bean tacos with mango avocado salsa.

Continue with similar patterns throughout the month, ensuring a diverse range of nutrient-dense foods to promote general health and well-being.

This meal plan focuses on complete foods, lean meats, healthy fats, and plenty of fruits and vegetables to help sarcoidosis patients improve their immune function and reduce inflammation. Individuals with sarcoidosis should speak with a healthcare expert or trained dietitian to receive personalized dietary recommendations based on their unique needs and preferences.

In closing the "Sarcoidosis Management Diet Cookbook," is vital to emphasize the importance of nutrition in assisting people with sarcoidosis in managing their symptoms and improving their general health. This cookbook has been painstakingly prepared to provide a collection of delicious and healthy recipes specifically adapted to the dietary requirements of those living with sarcoidosis.

Throughout this cookbook, we've emphasized the necessity of including anti-inflammatory foods, nutrient-dense components, and balanced meals to help decrease sarcoidosis symptoms and boost overall health. From delectable soups and robust salads to filling main dishes and healthy snacks, each recipe has been painstakingly created to not only satisfy the taste senses but also supply critical nutrients and enhance immunological function.

Furthermore, we've included a detailed 30-day meal plan to help readers incorporate these recipes into their daily lives. This meal plan emphasizes variety, balance, and portion control, ensuring that people with sarcoidosis get a wide range of nutrients while eating delicious and enjoyable meals all month.

As people deal with sarcoidosis, it's important to realize that dietary management is just one component of a holistic treatment plan. We encourage readers to collaborate with healthcare professionals, such as physicians and registered dietitians, to create personalized nutritional plans that address their unique needs and interests.

Finally, the "Sarcoidosis Management Diet Cookbook" is an invaluable resource for those living with sarcoidosis, providing practical advice, delicious recipes, and evidence-based nutritional information to help them on their journey to better health and well-being. Individuals with sarcoidosis can improve

their quality of life by leveraging the power of
nutrition.

THE END